Clinical Management of Hip Arthroplasty

Hartmuth Kiefer
Sylvia Usbeck
Leslie F. Scheuber
Volker Atzrodt

Clinical Management of Hip Arthroplasty

Practical Guide for the Use of Ceramic Implants

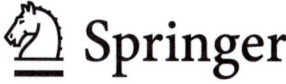

Hartmuth Kiefer MD, PhD
Clinic for Trauma and Orthopaedic Surgery
Hand and Reconstructive Surgery
Joint Center, Bünde
Akademisches Lehrkrankenhaus der MH Hannover
Hindenburgstraße 56, 32257 Bünde

Sylvia Usbeck
Leslie F. Scheuber
Volker Atzrodt PhD
CeramTec GmbH
CeramTec Platz 1–9
D-73207 Plochingen

ISBN 978-3-662-45491-6   ISBN 978-3-662-45492-3 (eBook)
DOI 10.1007/978-3-662-45492-3

Springer Medizin
© Springer-Verlag Berlin Heidelberg 2014
This work is subject to copyright. All rights are reserved by the Publisher, whether the whole
or part of the material is concerned, specifically the rights of translation, reprinting, reuse
of illustrations, recitation, broadcasting, reproduction on microfilms or in any other physical
way, and transmission or information storage and retrieval, electronic adaptation, computer
software, or by similar or dissimilar methodology now known or hereafter developed. Exempted
from this legal reservation are brief excerpts in connection with reviews or scholarly analysis or
material supplied specifically for the purpose of being entered and executed on a computer
system, for exclusive use by the purchaser of the work. Duplication of this publication or parts
thereof is permitted only under the provisions of the Copyright Law of the Publisher's location,
in its current version, and permission for use must always be obtained from Springer. Permissions for use may be obtained through RightsLink at the Copyright Clearance Center. Violations
are liable to prosecution under the respective Copyright Law.

The use of general descriptive names, registered names, trademarks, service marks, etc. in this
publication does not imply, even
in the absence of a specific statement, that such names are exempt from the relevant protective
laws and regulations and therefore free for general use. While the advice and information in
this book are believed to be true and accurate at the date of publication, neither the authors nor
the editors nor the publisher can accept any legal responsibility for any errors or omissions that
may be made. The publisher makes no warranty, express or implied, with respect to the material
contained herein.

Planning: Carola Herzberg
Cover Design: deblik Berlin
Cover Illustration: © Sebastian Kaulitzki, Fotolia
Production: Fotosatz-Service Köhler GmbH – Reinhold Schöberl, Würzburg

Printed on acid-free paper

Springer Medizin is brand of Springer
Springer is part of Springer Science+Business Media (www.springer.com)

Preface

The main goal of a well-designed, quality implant is to provide patients with a properly functioning device that restores the patient's quality of life.

Despite similarities, however, highest-quality implants are specifically designed according to manufacturers specifications and thus have to be implanted according to instructions provided by them. Don't mix and match is one of the basic rules. To avoid handling errors, it is of utmost importance that the surgeon follows a number of procedures that adhere to manufacturer's instructions and exacting criteria based on controlled study data to successfully implant the device. Since new data influence the surgical theater daily and the surgeon learns from her/his experience and that of others, the results are continuous modifications and corrections of actions. Training and know-how are essential prerequisites for the physician in charge. Ideally, the surgeon should be certified to avoid failure, most of which can be traced back to handling mistakes. Another part of the process should include an error analysis, in which the surgeon engages in reflection and continuous self assessment to analyzed her/his actions and the results. The error analysis provides new insights all the time which should lead to modifications of actions.

This pocket guide was written for orthopedic surgeons, who want to get informed quickly and thoroughly. The booklet was created as a guide, containing valuable tips for handling of ceramic implants in primary care. It renders expert information in a condensed form. The pocket guide is intended as a helpful teaching instrument that provides tips and tricks and deals with processes that prevent perfect outcomes. It was also written for the surgeon's own safety, to avoid claims and law suits after surgery. It is a guide from experienced clinicians for other clinicians, whether inexperienced or advanced.

Hartmuth Kiefer

Author

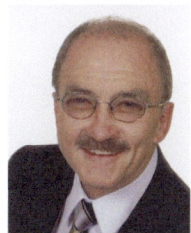

Hartmuth Kiefer, MD, PhD
Head of Orthopaedic and Trauma Department, Lukas Hospital Buende, Germany

Hartmuth Kiefer was born on Nov. 21, 1948, in Herrenberg, Germany, and studied medicine in Tübingen, Germany, and Innsbruck and Vienna, Austria. After becoming a surgeon, he became a specialist in orthopedic and trauma surgery and in sports medicine and physical therapy.

Hartmuth Kiefer
— served as a clinician
— has experience in teaching
— published 182 scientific papers, either as articles in scientific journals or as chapters in books
— and in addition worked as a court consultant (in Munich, Augsburg, Essen, Dortmund, etc.)

Kiefer performed his first endoprothesis in 1980. During his medical career – more than 20 years at Lukas – Kiefer has implanted more than 1,000 ceramic-on ceramic bearings each year. As a guest surgeon, he further introduced innovative surgical techniques to others in institutions outside of Lukas Hospital. In 1998, computer-navigated surgery was introduced in Bünde for knee endoprothesis and then was implemented for hip replacement in 2001. Currently all primary joint arthroplasties are navigated.

Kiefer is an internationally renown speaker and has presented more than 40 worldwide lectures and workshops since 2003. He currently is a member of numerous German societies for surgery and trauma surgery, such as the DGU, DGOOC and DGOU, as well as the European Society of Sports Traumatology, Knee Surgery and Arthroscopy (ESSKA), the American Academy of Orthopaedic Surgeons (AAOS) and the Societé Internationale de Chirugie Orthopédique et de Traumatologie (SICOT).

Table of Content

	Clinical Management of Hip Arthroplasty	1
	Practical Guide for the Use of Ceramic Implants	
	Hartmuth Kiefer, Sylvia Usbeck, Leslie F. Scheuber, Volker Atzrodt	
1	**Introduction**	2
2	**Compatibility of Implants**	2
3	**OR Planning and Choice of Implant**	4
4	**Ceramic Femoral Ball Head**	4
4.1	Protective Taper Cap	4
4.2	Careful Cleaning and Drying of the Stem Taper	6
4.3	Taper Locking	6
4.4	Positioning and Fixation of the Femoral Ball Head	9
4.5	Repositioning	11
5	**Ceramic Insert**	13
5.1	Versions	13
5.2	Cup Positioning	13
6	**Removal of Osteophytes**	14
7	**Functional Check with Trial Insert and Trial Femoral Ball Head**	16
8	**Positioning and Impaction of the Ceramic Insert**	17
9	**Summary**	20
	References	21

Clinical Management of Hip Arthroplasty

Practical Guide for the Use of Ceramic Implants

Hartmuth Kiefer, Sylvia Usbeck, Leslie F. Scheuber, Volker Atzrodt

1	Introduction	– 2
2	Compatibility of Implants	– 2
3	OR Planning and Choice of Implant	– 4
4	Ceramic Femoral Ball Head	– 4
4.1	Protective Taper Cap	– 4
4.2	Careful Cleaning and Drying of the Stem Taper	– 6
4.3	Taper Locking	– 6
4.4	Positioning and Fixation of the Femoral Ball Head	– 9
4.5	Repositioning	– 11
5	Ceramic Insert	– 13
5.1	Versions	– 13
5.2	Cup Positioning	– 13
6	Removal of Osteophytes	– 14
7	Functional Check with Trial Insert and Trial Femoral Ball Head	– 16
8	Positioning and Impaction of the Ceramic Insert	– 17
9	Summary	– 20
	References	– 21

1 Introduction

Ceramic implants (BIOLOX, CeramTec, Plochingen) have become established as the accepted standard of treatment for hip arthroplasty because of the outstanding outcomes associated with their use. Over the last four decades more than 10 million ceramic implants have been implanted worldwide. Today there is consensus that the problem of osteolysis induced by wear particles can be resolved effectively using ceramic femoral ball heads in articulation with ceramic and polyethylene inserts.

However, there is still much analysis and discussion of cases of failure based on clinical examples in the specialist literature. Complications are attributed to avoidable errors in the preoperative planning and use of the implants, and as a result recommendations for handling ceramic implants have been developed. Clinical experience has shown that complications [4][10][12][15][16][18][19][28] due to planning and handling can largely be avoided using suitable training and education measures.

Implant manufacturers provide surgeons with instructions for use and operating room (OR) manuals for the implants. These sources of advice are also intended to provide surgeons with valuable tips and tricks to safely handle ceramic implants illustrated with ample photographs from clinical practice.

2 Compatibility of Implants

Implants have designs specific to each manufacturer, and despite similar size information or taper labels, e.g., they have different angles, taper lengths (◘ Fig. 1), or insert designs.

Instructions for use from implant manufacturers provide information on which implants can be combined with others. This information must be heeded for technical reasons and because of liability and medical device law issues. Unapproved combinations of implant components may lead to complications and premature failure of the implants (◘ Fig. 2) [8][9][10][18][19][21][25][27]. To avoid such problems, implants from one manufacturer must not be combined with implants from others ("never mix and match"). In case of doubt, it is advisable to contact the manufacturer.

> **Take-Home Message**
>
> ☑ Implant geometry is always specific to a particular manufacturer.
> ☑ Follow the instructions for use provided by the implant manufacturer.
> ☒ Do not combine implant components from different manufacturers.
> ☒ There is no "Eurotaper" or 12/14 standard taper.
> ☒ There is no standardized external geometry for ceramic inserts.

2 · Compatibility of Implants

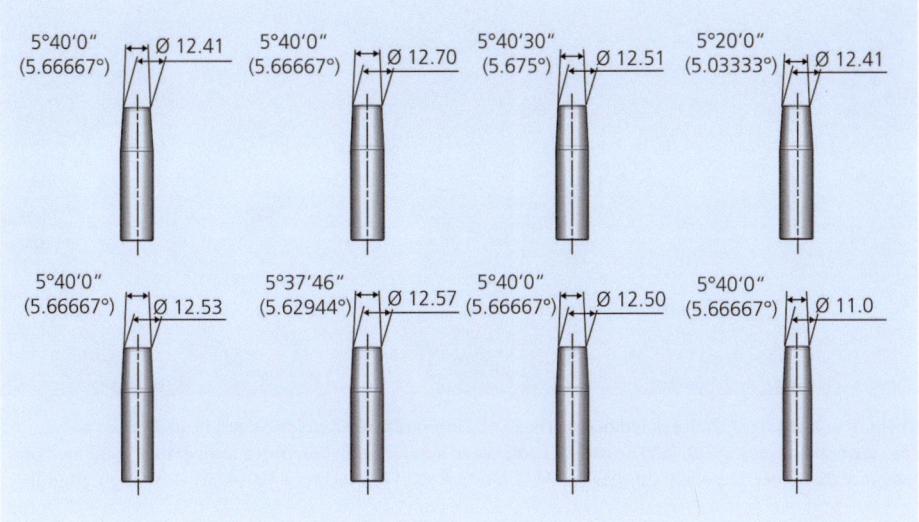

Fig. 1 Different tapers all of which are designated. 12/14 (Source: CeramTec)

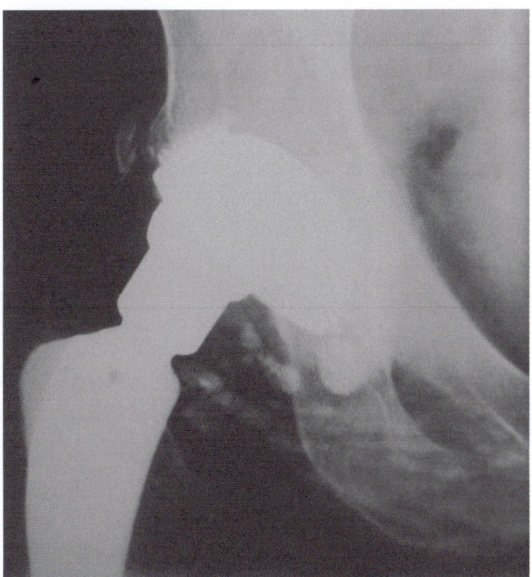

Fig. 2 Unapproved combination of a metal femoral ball head with a ceramic insert as a result of insufficient preoperative planning. This led to excessive wear of the metal femoral ball head, massive loss of metal, and premature failure of the implant. (Source: CeramTec)

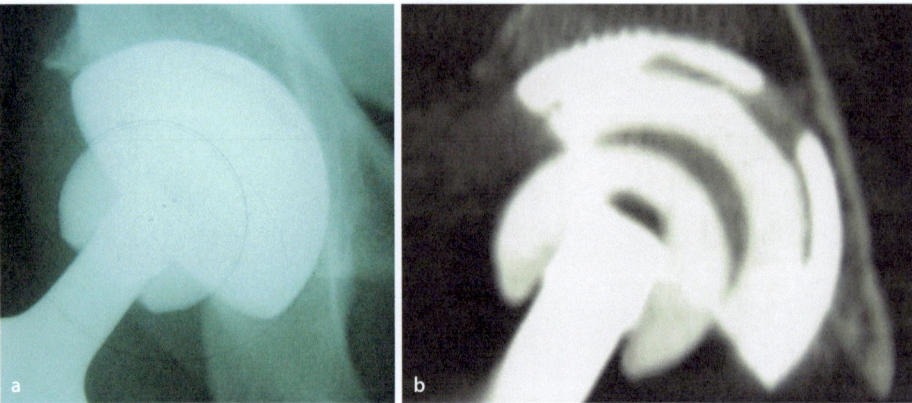

Fig. 3 a, b Incorrect choice of femoral ball head and insert diameter, which cannot be easily seen on the conventional radiograph (**a**). The patient complained about noises. Computed tomography confirmed the incorrect choice of component (**b**). (Source: M.M. Morlock MD, PhD, Technical University Hamburg-Harburg)

3 OR Planning and Choice of Implant

Careful preoperative planning is an essential prerequisite for choosing the correct components in terms of compatibility and size, offset, leg length correction, and positioning of the stem and cup relative to one another. Choosing the wrong components can lead to premature failure of the implant (Fig. 3a, b).

Take-Home Message
☑ Preoperative planning.

4 Ceramic Femoral Ball Head

4.1 Protective Taper Cap

The protective taper cap must not be removed too soon to avoid mechanical damage to the stem taper by instruments or other objects (Fig. 4a, b). Damage to the taper surface may lead to insufficient locking of the stem taper or stress concentrations developing in the internal taper of the femoral ball head.

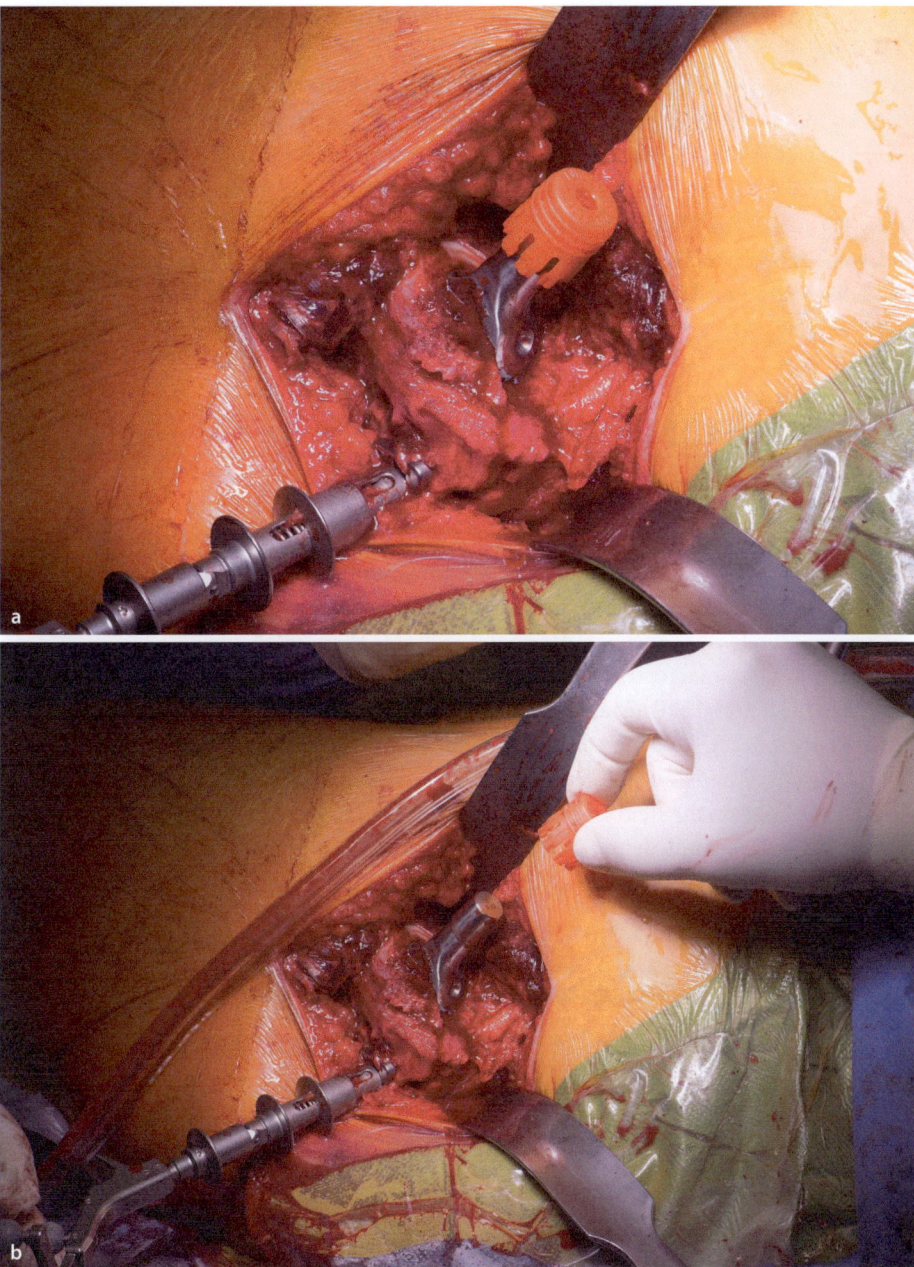

Fig. 4 **a** Protective taper cap. **b** Removing the protective taper cap

4.2 Careful Cleaning and Drying of the Stem Taper

As well as damage to the stem taper, contamination of the contact surfaces with foreign material (tissue, cement, bone, blood, etc.) affects the transfer of force to the ceramic femoral ball head and has a negative impact on the fracture strength of the femoral ball head (◘ Fig. 5) [22][23][24]. This means that it is essential to thoroughly clean and dry the stem taper (◘ Fig. 6, ◘ Fig. 7) intraoperatively after removing the protective taper cap (◘ Fig. 4b) and immediately prior to positioning of the femoral ball head. This is followed by another visual inspection of the stem taper for possible damage and contamination with foreign material (◘ Fig. 8).

4.3 Taper Locking

For modular hip arthroplasty it is necessary to join the ceramic femoral ball head and the stem taper intraoperatively. A secure connection prevents possible loosening of the femoral ball head as a result of friction forces in the joint. Secure taper locking ensures that relative movements between the components are avoided and the possibility of stem-side corrosion and release of metal particles and ions [11] is excluded.

The stem taper macrostructure has surface roughness (◘ Fig. 9).

When the femoral ball head is positioned on the stem taper, the structured taper surface deforms irreversibly. This increases the contact area and extrafrictional surfaces reinforce the torsional resistance of the femoral ball head. After the initial fixation of a ceramic femoral ball head on the stem taper, the taper surface of the stem is permanently deformed. For this reason, a ceramic femoral ball head must not be repositioned on such a stem taper.

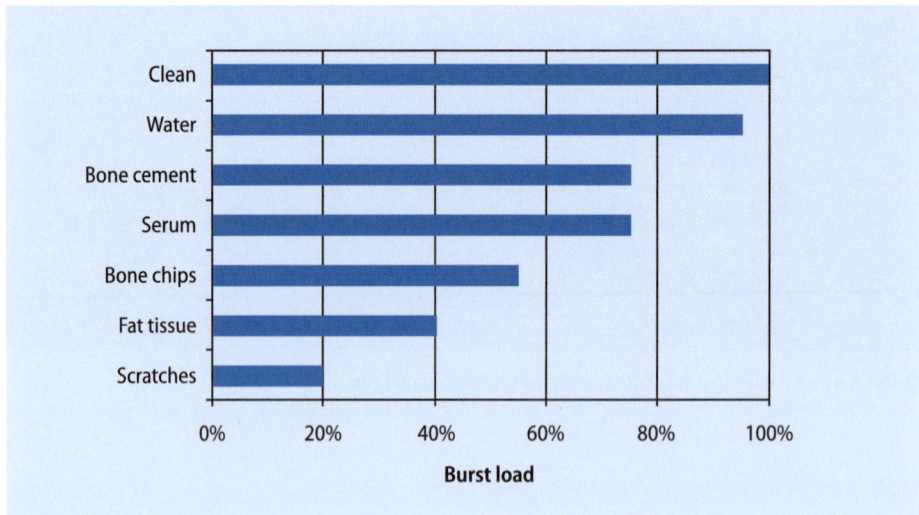

◘ Fig. 5 Contamination of the stem taper and effect on the burst load [22][23]. (Source: CeramTec)

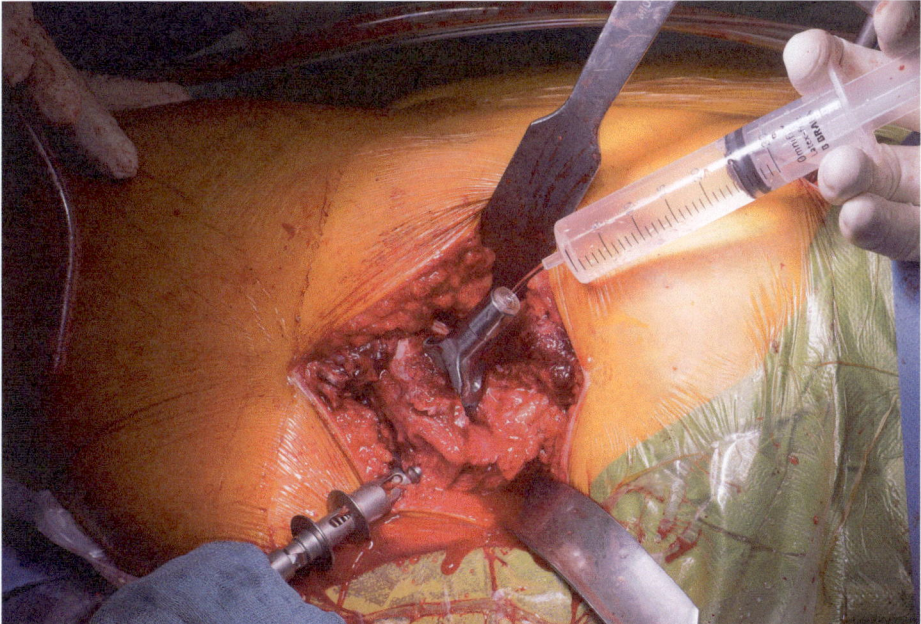

Fig. 6 Rinsing the stem taper

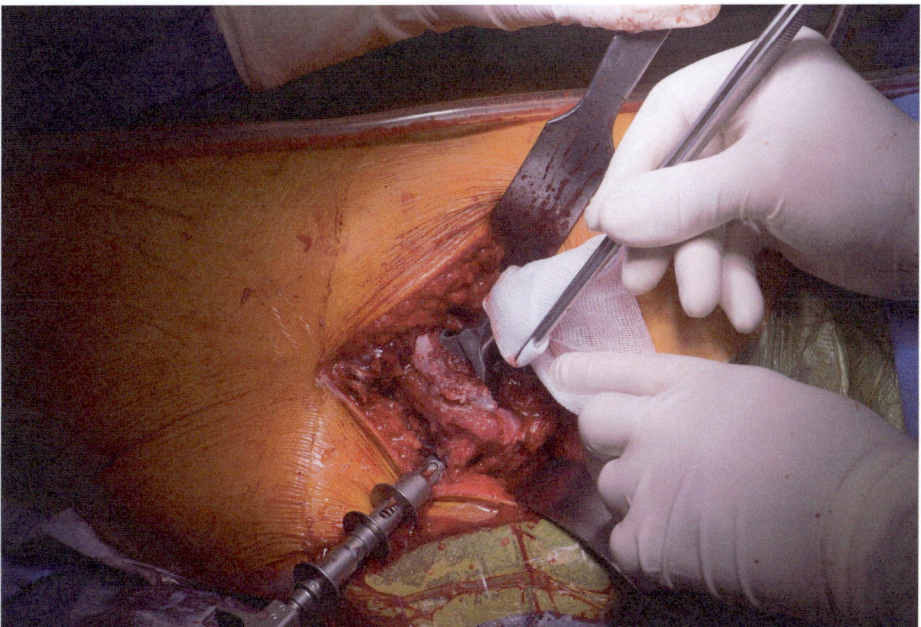

Fig. 7 Drying the stem taper

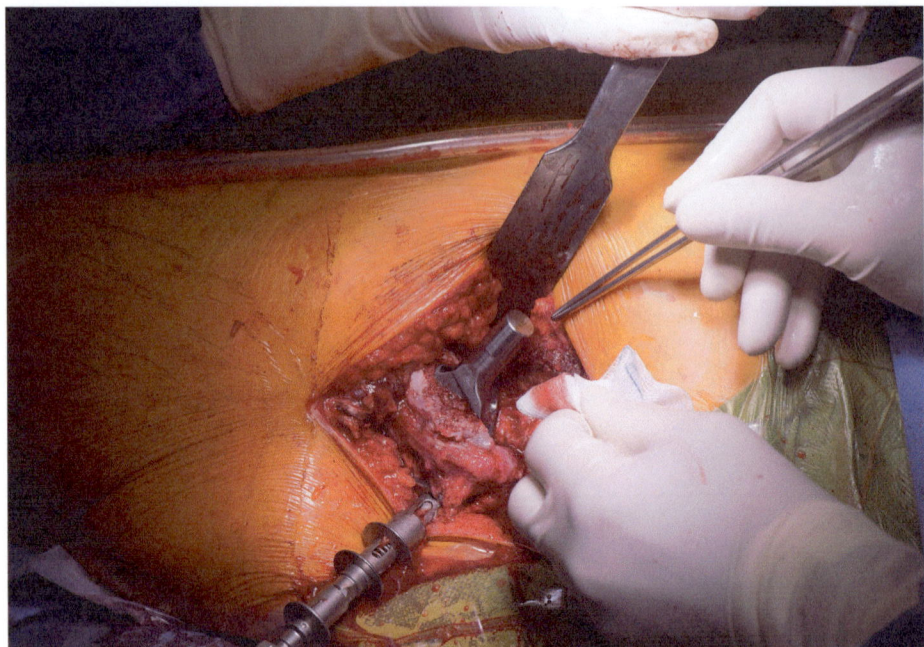

Fig. 8 After rinsing and drying, additional visual inspection of the stem taper for possible damage and contamination with foreign material

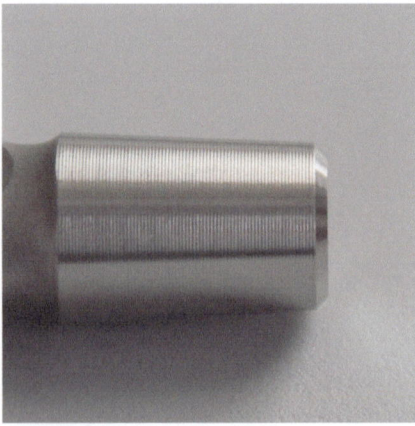

Fig. 9 Stem taper with grooved surface

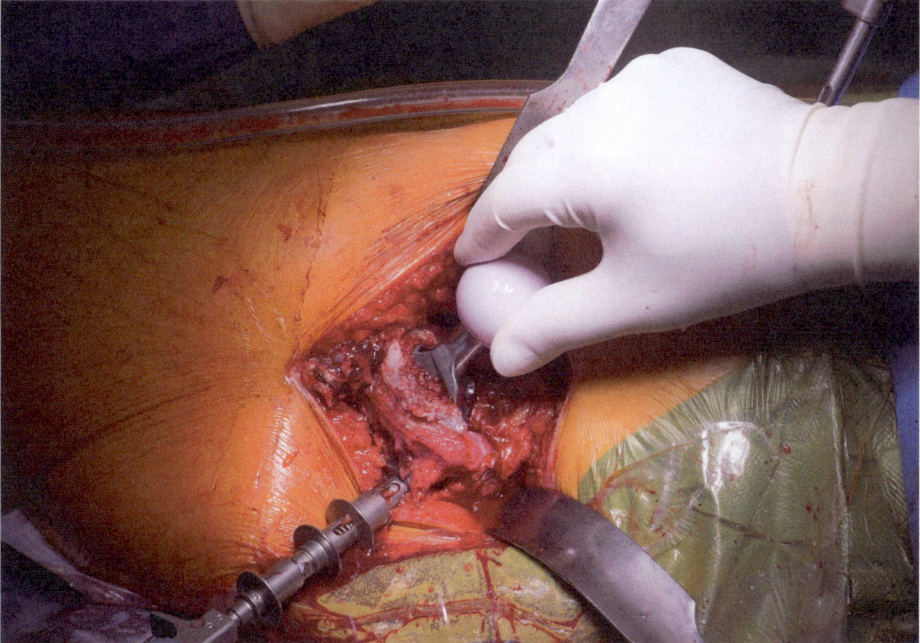

Fig. 10 Positioning the femoral ball head in the axial direction

If necessary, a ceramic revision femoral ball head specifically approved for this situation must be used in accordance with the instructions for use (ifu) of the implant manufacturer.

4.4 Positioning and Fixation of the Femoral Ball Head

The femoral ball head (Fig. 10) is positioned in the axial direction of the stem taper using a slight turning motion (Fig. 11) on the clean and dry stem taper.

After correctly positioning the femoral ball head, it is essential that the femoral ball head is locked with the stem taper. Investigations have shown that positioning the femoral ball head without additional impacting is not sufficient for a secure lock between the femoral ball head and the stem taper [22][23][24]. Using a moderate hammer blow on the impactor in the axial direction of the stem taper will ensure the femoral ball head is seated firmly (Fig. 12). A single hammer blow is sufficient, although several blows are permitted. Never strike the ceramic femoral ball head directly with a metal hammer so as to avoid damage (Fig. 13). Only the plastic head impactor provided by the respective endoprosthesis manufacturers must be used for this purpose.

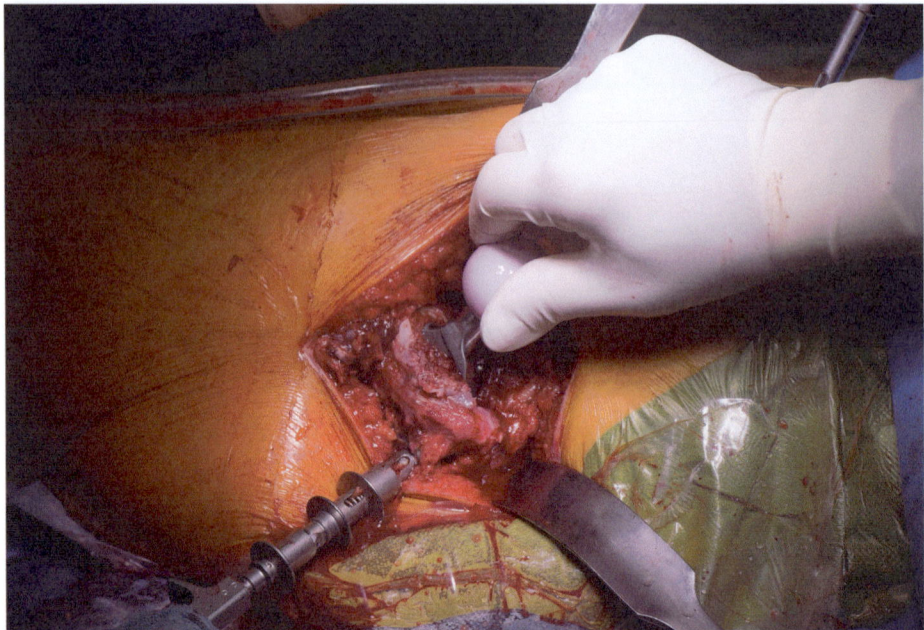

Fig. 11 Slight turning motion when positioning the femoral ball head

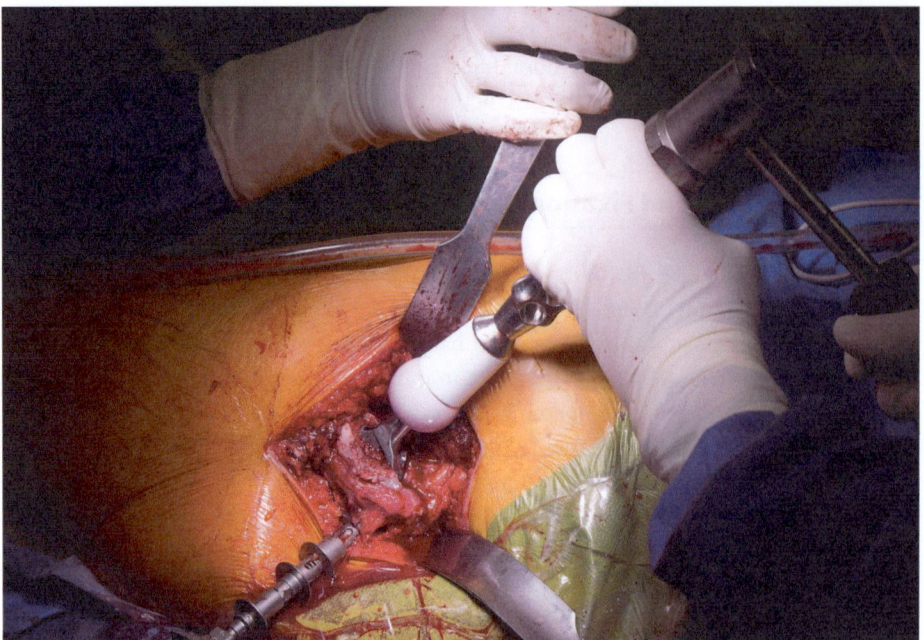

Fig. 12 Impacting the femoral ball head with a suitable instrument

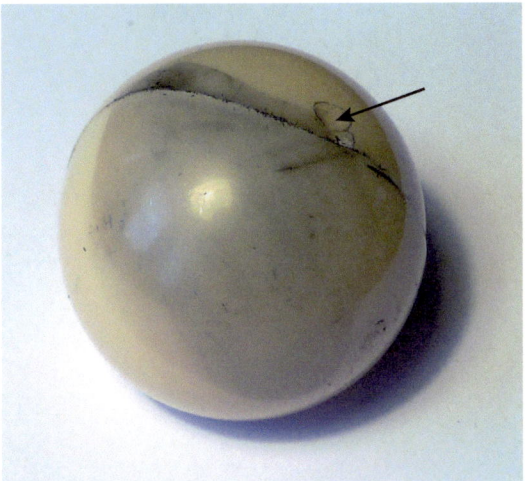

◘ **Fig. 13** Damage to the femoral ball head due to improper impaction (blow with a metal hammer directly to the femoral ball head). (With kind permission of M.M. Morlock MD, PhD, Technical University Hamburg-Harburg)

4.5 Repositioning

Prior to the final repositioning, the practice repositioning must be done using the trial femoral ball head with a simultaneous check of the range of movement (◘ Fig. 14). Once the functional check is complete, the trial femoral ball head has to be removed. The ceramic femoral ball head has to be positioned in the previously described manner. During the final repositioning, contact between the femoral ball head and metal (cup, instruments) must be avoided (◘ Fig. 15). Metal transfer can lead to an increase in the roughness of the ceramic surface and thus to a deterioration in the tribological properties [2][3][6][7][11][13][14][18][20][26][29][30]. After the repositioning (◘ Fig. 16), the functional check has to be repeated.

> **Take-Home Message**
>
> - ☑ Use a protective taper cap.
> - ☑ Keep the femoral ball head and stem taper clean and dry.
> - ☑ Position the femoral ball head using a turning motion while keeping it centered.
> - ☑ *Final* fixation of the femoral ball head using **only** the plastic impactor.
> - ☑ Single hammer blow is sufficient although several blows are permitted.
> - ☑ Practice repositioning with a check of the range of movement.
> - ☒ Do not remove the protective taper cap too soon.
> - ☒ Avoid metal transfer to the femoral ball head.
> - ☒ Never strike the femoral ball head directly with a metal hammer.

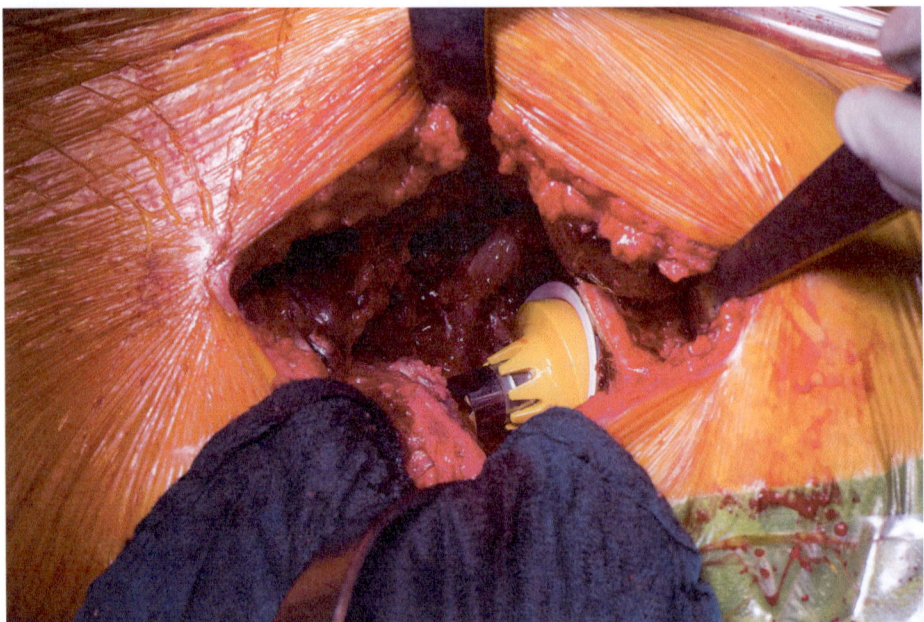

Fig. 14 Practice repositioning with the trial femoral ball head

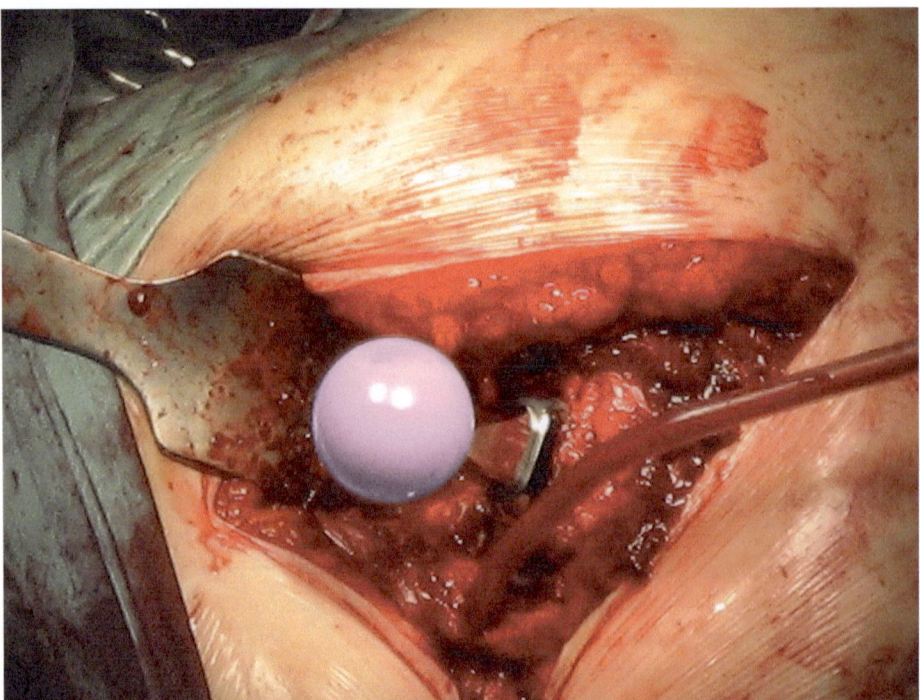

Fig. 15 Contact between the femoral ball head and metal instruments must be avoided during final repositioning. (Source: CeramTec)

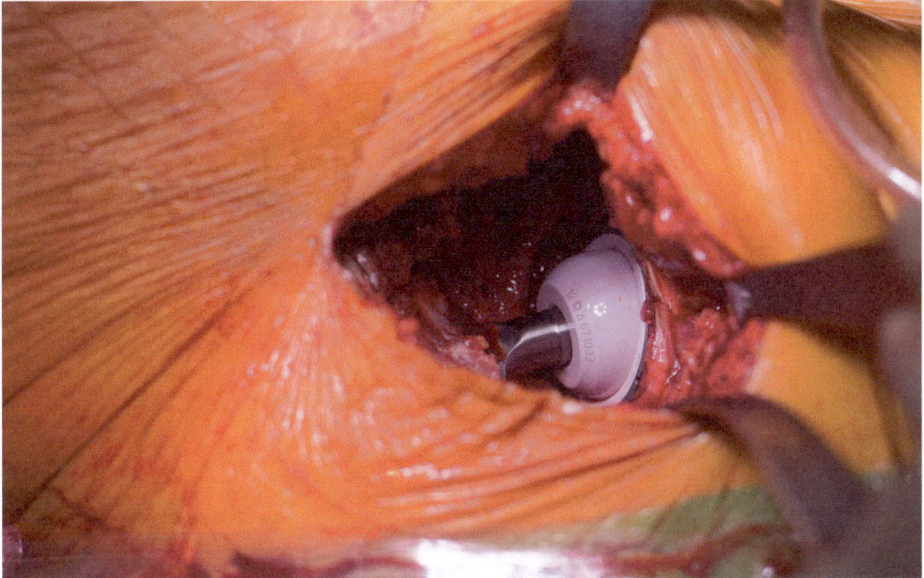

◘ **Fig. 16** Repositioning

5 Ceramic Insert

5.1 Versions

Ceramic inserts are fixed components of leading cup systems. In addition to the widespread modular systems, some manufacturers also offer premounted cup systems in which metal cups and ceramic inserts are already connected in the factory using a special procedure.

Modular premounted and mounted monoblock systems have the advantage of largely avoiding possible handling-related complications that may occur during intraoperative positioning of a ceramic insert, leading in turn to a reduction in the rate of complications [5].

5.2 Cup Positioning

To achieve the best possible range of motion and to avoid impingement [1], the cup must be positioned in the safe zone as defined by Lewinnek [17] (◘ Fig. 17). This means that the inclination of the cup should not greatly exceed or fall below a value of 40–45°. The same also applies to the anteversion of the cup. In this case, the value should not greatly exceed or fall below 10–20°. If these ranges are not adhered to, it can lead to subluxations and/or dislocations of the femoral ball head out of the ceramic insert. With a cup position outside these values, a ceramic insert must not be used.

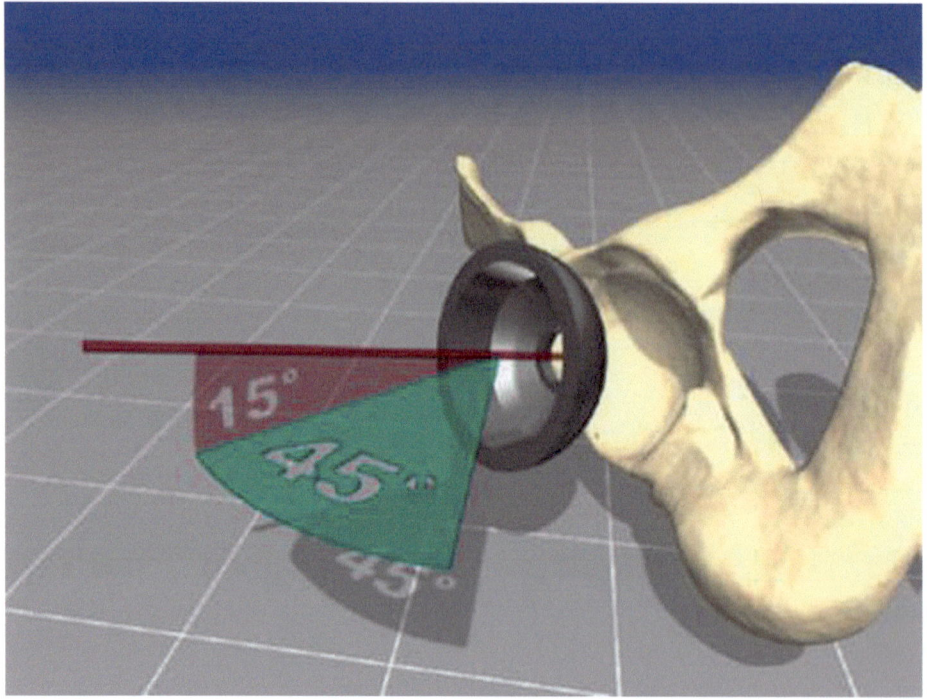

Fig. 17 Cup positioning within the Lewinnek safe zone. (Source: CeramTec/Paracam)

For cups that are placed in a retroverted position, a ceramic insert must not be used. This may otherwise lead to nonphysiological force transmissions (increased contact pressure) on the cup rim, which is associated with increased ceramic wear.

Take-Home Message

- ☑ Position the cup in the Lewinnek safe zone.
- ☒ Do *not* use ceramic inserts with retroverted cups.

6 Removal of Osteophytes

Osteophytes must be removed (Fig. 18a, b) to avoid impingement.

Take-Home Message

- ☑ Remove osteophytes.

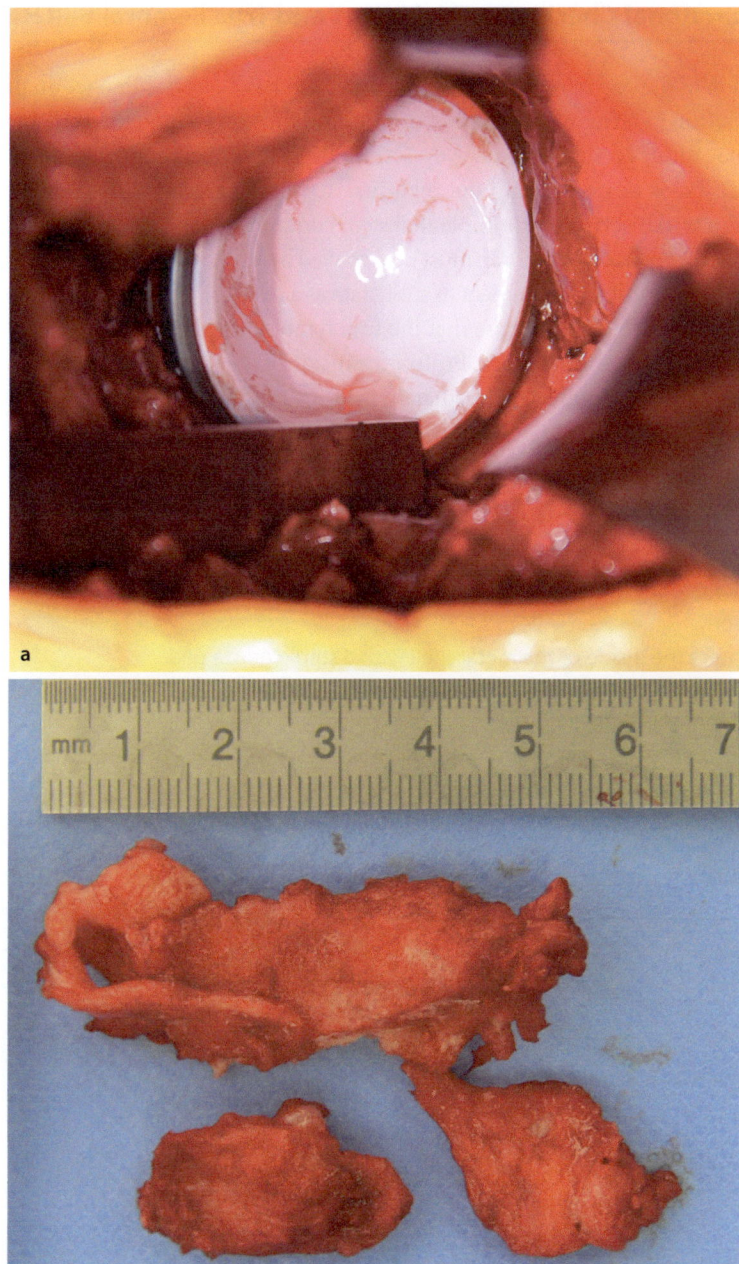

Fig. 18 a, b Removal of the osteophytes

7 Functional Check with Trial Insert and Trial Femoral Ball Head

The position of the cup in relation to the implant stem has a direct influence on the success of the operation in terms of the range of motion and thus on the potential risk of impingement, dislocation, or subluxation. Any screws used must be completely sunk into the metal shell. Prior to positioning the final insert, a complete functional check must be done using a trial insert with the implanted stem components and a trial femoral ball head (◘ Fig. 19). The protective taper cap must be removed before the functional check. The joint must not dislocate during movement or subluxate as a result of impingement of the implant components or soft tissues. Ensure that the trial femoral ball head and the trial insert are removed after the functional check. Protect the inside of the metal shell with a sterile gauze pad (◘ Fig. 20) and remove it immediately prior to the final positioning of the ceramic insert.

> **Take-Home Message**
>
> ☑ Functional check with trial femoral ball head and trial insert.
> ☑ After completing the functional check, remove trial femoral ball head and trial insert.
> ☑ Protect the inside of the metal shell with a sterile gauze pad.

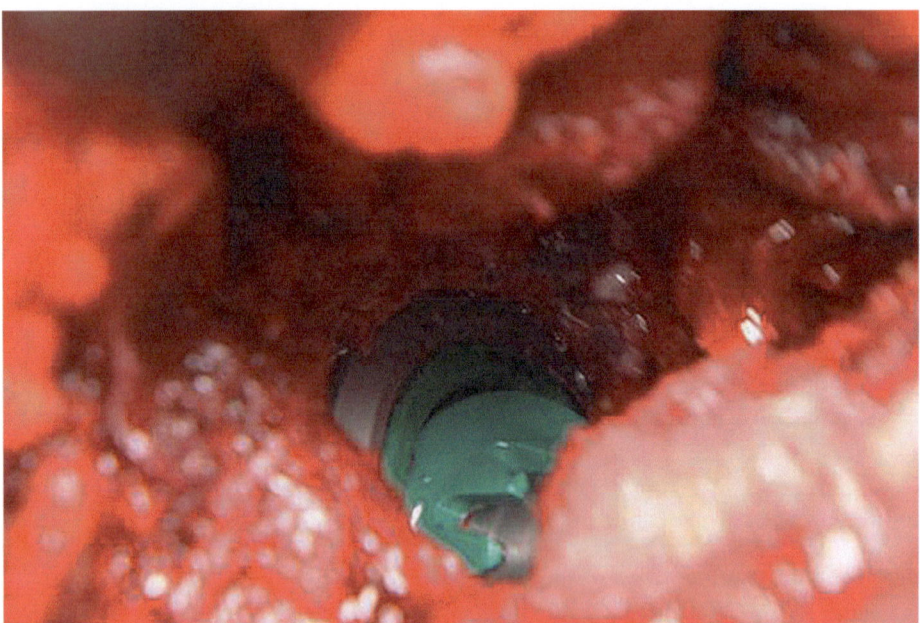

◘ Fig. 19 Functional check (with trial insert and trial femoral ball head)

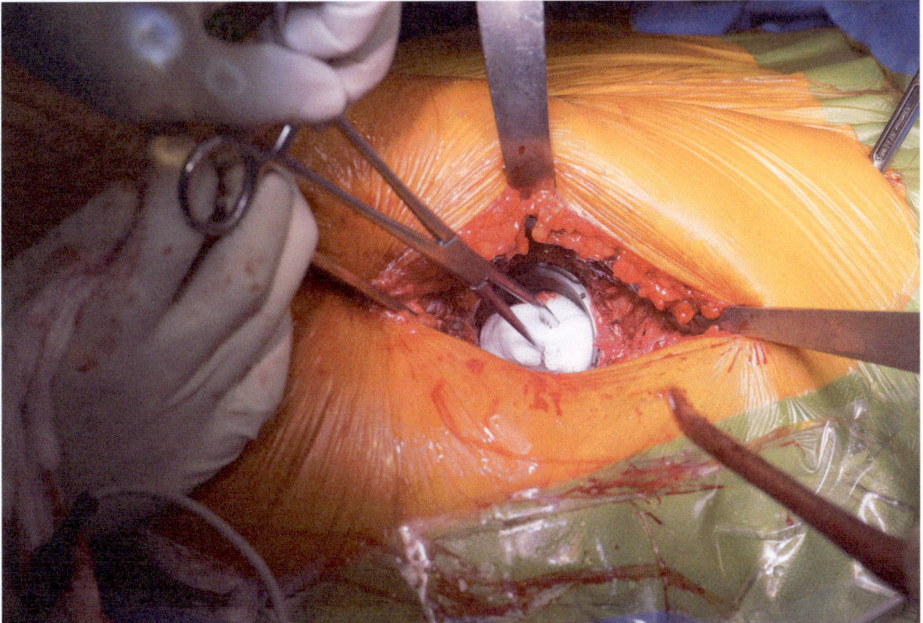

Fig. 20 Protection of the interior of the metal shell with a sterile gauze pad

8 Positioning and Impaction of the Ceramic Insert

Ceramic inserts require careful handling during positioning and impaction. Checking the correct seat of the ceramic insert in the metal shell is essential. The metal shell must be clean and dry prior to the ceramic insert being positioned. Fluids, fatty tissue, bone fragments, and traces of cement cannot be compressed (Fig. 5) and must be removed from the metal shell. Implant manufacturers provide positioning instruments that are used to avoid skewed positioning of the insert (Fig. 21a–c). When using a positioning instrument, follow the instructions for use provided by the manufacturer.

The correct seat of the ceramic insert in the metal shell is checked by feeling the cup rim with the finger (Fig. 22). The metal and ceramic rim must lie flush with one another (Fig. 23). If the ceramic insert is skewed or tilted, this can lead to the rim of the insert becoming chipped and damage to the metal shell [28]. The incorrectly positioned ceramic insert must be removed with instruments recommended by the endoprosthesis manufacturer. A ceramic insert that has been positioned and removed must not be reused. Due to the precise fit required between the ceramic insert and the metal shell, only new and undamaged components must be used. If the locking surface of the metal shell is damaged, a ceramic insert must not be used. For the final fitting of the ceramic insert, an impactor suitable for ceramic inserts and recommended by the prosthesis company is used to firmly position it with a slight hammer stroke in the axial direction (Fig. 24). Never strike the ceramic insert directly with a metal hammer.

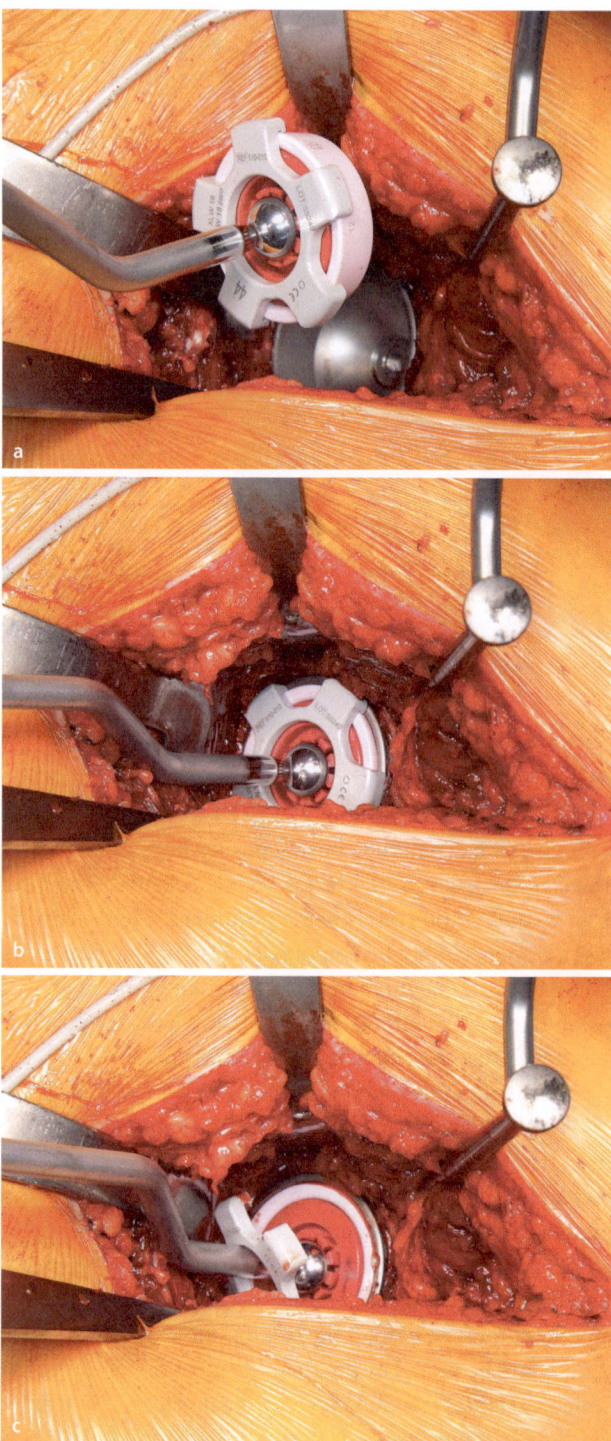

Fig. 21 a–c Positioning instrument in clinical use (example)

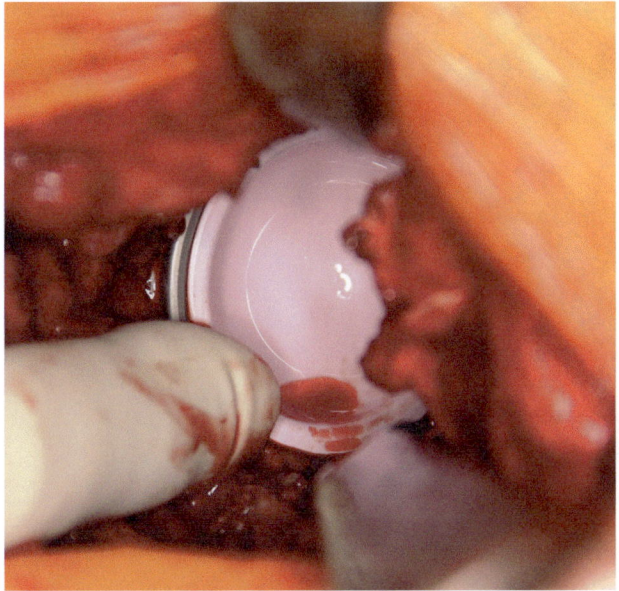

Fig. 22 Manually feeling the cup rim

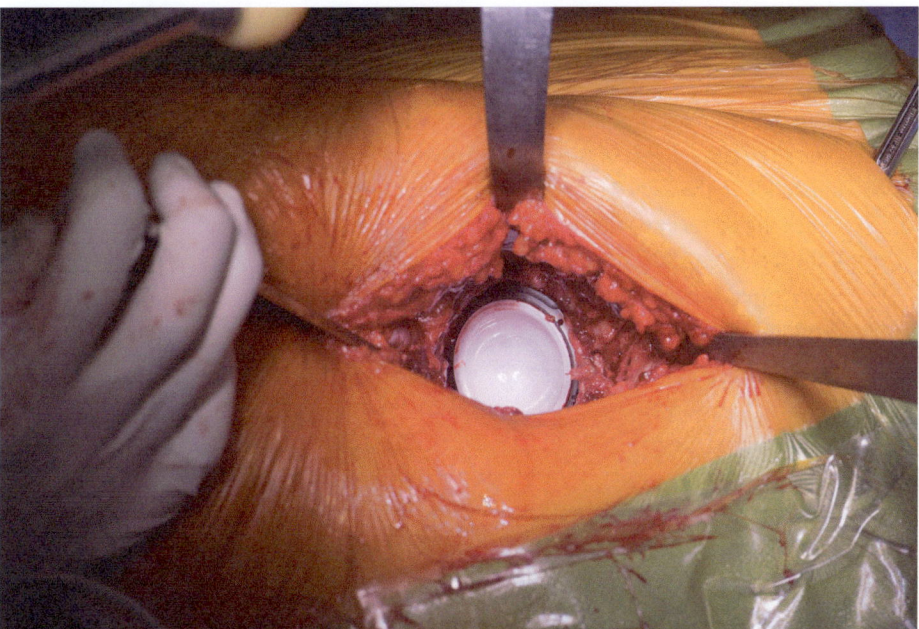

Fig. 23 The metal and ceramic rim must lie flush with one another

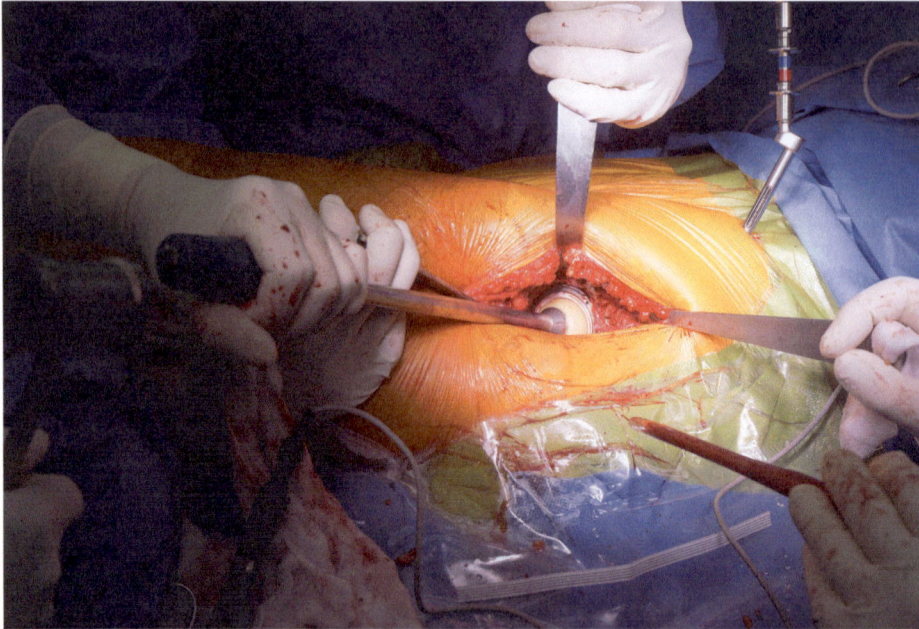

Fig. 24 Impaction of the ceramic insert

Take-Home Message

- ☑ Keep the ceramic insert and cup clean and dry.
- ☑ Check the correct seat of the insert by manually feeling the cup rim.
- ☑ Impaction in the axial direction using a suitable impactor.
- ☑ Check the correct position of the insert in the metal shell (radiographic check).
- ☒ If the locking surface on the metal shell is damaged, do not use a ceramic insert.
- ☒ An incorrectly positioned ceramic insert must be removed.
- ☒ A ceramic insert that has been positioned and removed must not be reused.
- ☒ Do not combine implant components from different manufacturers.

9 Summary

All implant materials may lead to adverse results such as increased wear under certain conditions. Important influencing factors for unimpaired long-term function of the hip arthroplasty include precise operative planning, intraoperative realization of the correct position of the stem and cup, and careful handling of all components. If the criteria regarding implant design, implant position, and handling of components are all met, ceramic implants can significantly reduce wear-related loosening. This has been verified by the excellent clinical results achieved with ceramic implants over a period of more than 40 years.

References

1. Bader R, Willmann G (1999) Ceramic cups for hip endoprostheses, 6: Cup design, inclination and antetorsion angle modify range of motion and impingement [German]. Biomed Tech (Berl) 44(7-8):212–219
2. Bal BS, Rahaman MN, Aleto T, Miller FS, Traina F, Toni A (2005) Surface changes to alumina femoral heads after metal staining during implantation, and after recurrent dislocations of the prosthetic hip. In: D'Antonio J, Dietrich M (eds) Ceramics and alternative bearings in joint arthroplasty. Steinkopff Verlag, Darmstadt, pp 147–154
3. Bal BS, Rahaman MN, Aleto T, Miller FS, Traina F, Toni A (2007) The significance of metal staining on alumina femoral heads in total hip arthroplasty. J Arthroplasty 22:14–19
4. Callanan MC, Jarrett B, Bragdon CR, Zurakowski D, Rubash HE, Freiberg AA, Malchau H (2011) The John Charnley Award: risk factors for cup malpositioning: quality improvement through a joint registry at a tertiary hospital. Clin Orthop Relat 469:319–329
5. CeraNews (2012) Complication rate of ceramic components – an update, 2:16–219
6. Chang CB, Yoo JJ, Song WS, Kim DJ, Koo KH, Kim HJ (2008) Transfer of metallic debris from the metal surface of an acetabular cup to artificial femoral heads by scraping: comparison between alumina and cobalt-chrome heads. J Biomed Mater Res B Appl Biomater 85:204–209
7. Chevillotte C, Trousdale RT, An KN, Padgett D, Wright T (2012) Retrieval analysis of squeaking ceramic implants: Are there related specific features? Orthop Traumatol Surg Res 98:281–287
8. D'Antonio JA, Capello WN, Bierbaum B, Manley M, Naughton M (2006) Ceramic-on-ceramic bearings for total hip arthroplasty: 5-9 year follow-up. Semin Arthro 17:146–152
9. Hinrichs F, Griss P (2001). Retrieved wear couple ceramic-on-metal: A case study. In Toni A, Willmann G (eds) Bioceramics in joint arthroplasty. Georg Thieme Verlag, Stuttgart, New York, pp 99–102.
10. Hohman DW, Affonso J, Anders M (2011) Ceramic-on-ceramic failure secondary to head-neck taper mismatch. Am J Orthop 40(11):571–573
11. Isaac GH, Brockett C, Breckon A, van der Jagt D, Williams S, Hardaker C, Fisher J, Schepers A (2009) Ceramic-on-metal bearings in total hip replacement: whole blood metal ion levels and analysis of retrieved components. J Bone Joint Surg Br 91-B:1134–1141
12. Jeffers JRT, Walter WL (2012). Ceramic-on-ceramic bearings in hip arthroplasty. J Bone Joint Surg Br 94-B: 735–745
13. Kim YH (2007). Surface roughness of ceramic femoral heads after in vivo transfer of metal: correlation to polyethylene wear. In: Chang JD, Billau K (eds) Bioceramics and alternative bearings in joint arthroplasty. Steinkopff Verlag, Darmstadt, p 49
14. Kim YH, Ritchie A, Hardaker C (2005) Surface roughness of ceramic femoral heads after in vivo transfer of metal: correlation to polyethylene wear. J Bone Joint Surg Am 87:577–582
15. Kusaba A, Sunami H, Kondo S, Kuroki Y (2011) Uncemented Ceramic-on-ceramic bearing couple for dysplastic osteoarthritis: A 5-to 11-year follow-up study. Semin Arthro 22:240–247
16. Lee GC, Garino JP (2011) Reliability of ceramic components. Semin Arthroplasty 22:271–275
17. Lewinnek GE, Lewis JL, Tarr R, Compere CL, Zimmerman JR (1978). Dislocations after total hip-replacement arthroplasties. J Bone Joint Surg 60-A 2:217–20
18. Morlock MM, Huber H, Bishop N (2013) Technology and handling of ceramic implants. In: Knahr K (ed) Total hip arthroplasty. Tribological considerations and clinical consequences. Springer, Berlin Heidelberg New York, pp 3–16
19. Morlock M, Nassutt R, Janssen R, Willmann G, Honl M (2001) Mismatched wear couple zirconium oxide and aluminium oxide in total hip arthroplasty. J Arthroplasty 16(8):1071–1074
20. Muller FA, Hagymasi M, Greil P, Zeiler G, Schuh A (2006) Transfer of metallic debris after dislocation of ceramic femoral heads in hip prostheses. Arch Orthop Trauma Surg 126:174–180
21. Oldenburg M, Wegner R, Baur X (2009) Severe cobalt intoxication due to prosthesis wear in repeated total hip arthroplasty. J Arthroplasty 24(5):825e 15–20
22. Pandorf T (2010) the importance of clean taper conditions using ceramic hip implants. In: Cobb (ed) Modern trends in THA bearings, material and clinical performance. Springer, Berlin Heidelberg, New York, pp 97–102
23. Pandorf T, Hummes J, Preuss R (2008) Einfluss der Oberflächenqualität von Schaftkonen auf die Bruchkraft von keramischen Kugelköpfen (poster). Presented at the annual congress of the DKOU

24. Pandorf T, Preuss R, Czak R (2010) Impaction forces and proper seating of ceramic ball heads (poster). Presented at the annual meeting of the Orthopaedic Research Society (ORS)
25. Ratzel R, Rehborn M (2007) Unterschätztes Problem. Kombination von Komponenten verschiedener Hersteller bei der Hüftendoprothetik. Orthopädie im Profil 1:46–47
26. Schuh A, Holzwarth U, Kachler W, Gaske J, Zeiler G (2004). Titanauflagerungen auf Keramikköpfen bei luxierten Hüftendoprothesen. Der Orthopäde 33:1194–1200
27. Steens W, Foerster G, Katzer A (2006). Severe cobalt poisoning with loss of sight after ceramic-metal pairing in a hip – a case report. Acta Orthopaedica 77(5):830–832
28. Steinhauser E, Bader R, Mittelmeier W (2004) Schadensanalyse anhand zweier Fälle von Keramikbrüchen von Pfanneninserts. Empfehlungen zur Vermeidung handhabungsbedingter Brüche. [Damage analysis illustrated by two cases of broken ceramic inserts. Recommendations for avoiding breakages caused by handling.] Orthopäde 33:332–333
29. Tomek IM, Currier JH, Mayor MB, Van Citters DW (2012) Metal Transfer on a ceramic head with a single rim contact. J Arthroplasty 27(2):324.e–4
30. Weber S, Holzwarth U, Kachler W, Göske J, Zeiler G, Schuh A (2004) Titanauflagerungen auf Keramikköpfen in der Hüftendoprothetik [abstract]. Biomaterials 5:133

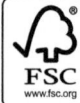

MIX
Papier aus verantwortungsvollen Quellen
Paper from responsible sources
FSC® C105338

If you have any concerns about our products,
you can contact us on
ProductSafety@springernature.com

In case Publisher is established outside the EU,
the EU authorized representative is:
**Springer Nature Customer Service Center GmbH
Europaplatz 3, 69115 Heidelberg, Germany**

Printed by Libri Plureos GmbH
in Hamburg, Germany